THE ASTROLOGICAL PHYSICIAN

ASTROLOGICAL MEDICINE

First Edition 1658
William Andrews

Modern English Edition 2017
Edited by Tarl Warwick

COPYRIGHT AND DISCLAIMER

PREFACE TO THE 2017 EDITION

This interesting work is a fine example of one of the primordial ideas that would later influence the whole of revolutionary-era science and spirituality. The (mostly) predictable movement of celestial bodies was assumed by those at the time to overlap with disease, since the humors as they envisioned them would surely, if their theories were true, be influenced by the planets and stars, with their vastness and spiritual overtones.

Thus this text admonishes the physician (at the time little more than an herbalist with a bloodletting device, alcohol, and a bag of star charts) to take note of the astronomical state at the time of a patients' complaints, giving an overview of the likely problem and the course of the disease- it even claims the ability to judge the chance of a patient dying or recovering. In a further, and perhaps in the most funny twist, it also proclaims the possibility of witchery or demons and suggests certain astrological situations which would indicate the likelihood of them.

This particular astrological medicine would fairly quickly lose favor to the more refined (and less certain) practice of fortune telling which was more likely to suggest the actual result; in some cases as good as a 50% chance, as opposed to an astrological system which contains dozens of total astrological situations to note.

This edition of the Astrological Physician has been edited from archaic 17th century English into modern English. Care has been taken to retain all original meaning.

THE ASTROLOGICAL PHYSICIAN

Showing how to find out the cause and nature of a disease, according to the secret rules of the art of ASTROLOGY

Also general rules and instructions, teaching how to discover what part of the body is afflicted

With a perfect description of the diseases and Infirmities, signified by the Planets, in any of the twelve Zodiacal Constellations, together with a most exact method, showing how to find whether the sick shall live or die, according to natural causes; with an exact way how to find the true Crisis, Judicial or Critical days.

Being of excellent use for all such as study Physic.

TO THE READER

Courteous Reader,

It is not the maliciousness of the present times, or the detracting tongues of men in this Critical Age, that shall hinder me from benefiting posterity with my labor; for although this peevish generation might justly cause me to bury my conceptions in silence and obscurity, yet in regard of the great affection I bear unto all those who are lovers of art and learning, I am induced to engage upon this subject: it were needless here to show what great necessity there is for every physician to be an astrologer, or to practice physic astrologically, in regard of the great influence and dominion the planets and stares have on our bodies, seeing no rational man can deny or disprove the same, although many have endeavored what they can to contradict the truth.

I confess many there are of men in these our times, which labor strongly to prove, if it were possible, by their many weak arguments, that the heavens have no power or influence on inferior things here below; these I answer, *Ars non habet inimicum, praeter ignorantem*, which indeed is really verified in these sort of men which deny the stars to have influence upon the inferior and elementary things, in regard ignorance causes this their foolish opinion but I shall leave these, and apply to the judicious and more sober spirited men, for whose sake I have composed this present work, that so I might benefit all those who desire to proceed in the study and practice of physic astrologically, whose kind accepting hereof shall animate me to acquaint posterity with my future labors.

In the present treatise, I have very briefly shown how to judge upon any disease or sickness whatsoever, and to find out and discover the nature, cause and quality thereof, according to the secret rules of astrology. I have also clearly shown the diseases and infirmities signified by the seven planets, by themselves, and by their several positions, in any of the twelve signs: I have further for the benefit of all astrological physicians, or any others, who desire to study physic astrologically, plainly, and very copiously shown how to discover what part of the body is afflicted, whether the sick be curable or not, or designed for life or death, according to natural causes; with exact rules how to discover the same; as also, a succinct method to judge, whether any fascination or witchcraft cause the sickness and distemper, or whether the disease be natural or not.

I have also shewed how to find the exact or true crisis, with the critical and judicial days, yet notwithstanding, I have not been so copious upon the discovery of the true crisis, as I doe intend hereafter (God willing) in another work.

If this small piece shall find your kind acceptation, it shall encourage me to prosecute my study in this kind, for your benefit and profit hereafter: In the meantime, if any carping critics shall be offended with me for this work, I shall not much value or regard their malice and envy, being already acquainted therewith, knowing the better how to bear it: I have no more at present to inform you of, but that I am your real friend more then you expect.

December 20, Anno Christi, 1655.
William Andrews

IN PRAISE OF THE ENSUING ASTROLOGICAL PHYSICIAN

Though the author of this treatise is wholly unknown unto me, yet. I could not but give this little book of his, and himself thus much commendations, namely, That he has judiciously performed the work in hand, with much brevity, and after a handsome and easy method, so that a reasonable understanding, after he can but truly erect a Scheme of Heaven by Hartgills Tables, may with much certainty discover by his rules here laid down, the cause and humor offending; his directions are short, plain and significant; he has deduced the diseases mankind is subject unto very rationally and naturally from each planet, so that any astrologer, if but meanly capable, may now by his industry receive infinite satisfaction. And the physicians of his age, how learned soever, need not disdain the perusal or practical part hereof, in regard of the great benefit, which from hence will accrue unto their patients, who many times die, ere the cause of their disease is made known, for neither the urine, pulse, or words of the sick, can so truly inform the doctor, as a right position of Heaven. *William Lilly, Student in Astrology.*

THE ASTROLOGICAL PHYSICIAN

In the first place for the basis or foundation of our work, we ought carefully to observe that moment of time (if it may be obtained) that the sick party was first oppressed with the disease, sickness or infirmity; but if the exact time cannot be obtained of the parties first falling sick, namely the year, day, hour and minute, then we ought to observe that very moment when the urine was first brought to the physician for his judgment thereon; but if no urine be brought then the very time must be accepted of, when first the physician speaks with the sick party, and then recourse being had to an Ephemeris or astronomical tables, let a figure of heaven be erected, and place the planets therein, especially the place of the Moon must be exactly rectified, because the crisis of diseases and critical days are found out by her motion; having erected a figure of heaven, observe what sign is in the ascendant or first house, what planet or planets are therein posited or aspecting the house, then have regard unto the Lord of the ascendent, and consider what sign he is in, and in what house he is posited, what planet or planets are in configuration with him, what houses they are lords of, whether fortunate or unfortunate, which being observed, have recourse to the sixth house, and lord thereof, and observe what sign descends on the cusps of that house, and what planet or planets are posited therein, and what planet or planets are in configuration with the lord thereof, and what aspect they have unto the ascendant, for from the sixth house and lord thereof, do we regard to the place of Moon and lord of the ascendant, and those planets placed therein, and the signs wherein they shall be found. require the nature and quality of any disease, or sickness, having regard to the place of the sun and lord of the ascendant, and those planets placed therein and the figures wherein they shall be found.

THE ASTROLOGICAL PHYSICIAN

If the Party be really sick for whom the question is propounded

For discovering whether the party be sick or not, we ought to consider, if that the ascendant and lord thereof be free from all manner of impediment, in other words, that no malevolent planet be posited in the ascendant, or in configuration with the lord thereof, or if any fixed star of the nature of the lord of the sixth house, or of the nature of Saturn, or Mars, or of the lords of the 8th, or 12th houses be in the ascendant, or with the lord thereof, and if Jupiter or Venus who be naturally fortuitous shall be in the first house, or with the lord thereof, and they not having any dignities in the sixth or 8th houses in the figure, and the lord of the ascendant essentially fortified, well posited in a good house of heaven, and not directly under the Suns' beams or retrograde, then the party is not sick, but is distempered with some accidental cause, which may suddenly be rectified: But howsoever the party is not naturally sick, but accidentally afflicted with some outward cause, for if the lord of the ascendant be free from all impediment, and in no aspect with the lords of the sixth or 8th houses, it is an assured testimony that nature is strong.

But on the contrary; if the ascendant shall be afflicted, or the Lord thereof out of his essential dignities retrograde, and afflicted by the unfortunate, or be in the sixth house, or the lord of the sixth in the ascendant, it is a strong argument the party for whom the question is demanded is really sick and diseased, so likewise if any fixed stars of the nature of the lord of the sixth house arise in the ascendant, or be with the lord thereof in a bad house of heaven, and they likewise of a malevolent nature intimate of the same.

THE ASTROLOGICAL PHYSICIAN

Of the Nature and quality of the disease or sickness

When we have found that the party is sick, we ought to discover the nature of the humor offending, or quality of the disease, which that we may doe, observe first what sign is in the sixth house, and what sign ascends in the first house, in what sign the Lords of those houses are in; which being well understood, will acquaint us with the nature of the disease, for if the lord of the sixth house shall be in fiery signs, they intimate the disease or sickness proceeds from choleric humors, and that choler abounds, so likewise if they shall be in watery signs, they declare that the cause of the disease proceeds from moist causes, and that the present distemper arises from the abundance of moist and watery humors; and so moreover, if that the lord of the ascendant, and the lord of the sixth house, and the Moon shall be in earthly signs, it intimates that the disease or sickness has its origin from melancholy, and that black and addust choler abound, and so likewise when they shall be posited in airy signs, they shew that the sickness or infirmity proceeds from corruption of blood, and that the blood is putrefied, for the lord of the ascendant, and lord of the sixth house, and Moon declares the nature and quality of the disease to be according to the nature of the sign, or triplicity they are in, for as they are the principal signs in a disease, so the sign wherein they are posited do in part show the nature of the disease of sickness; for as there are twelve signs in the Zodiac, so are the for elements governed and signified by the twelve signs, namely, Aries, Leo, Sagittarius rule the fiery triplicity, Gemini, Libra, Aquarius govern the Aiery triplicity. Taurus, Virgo, Capricorn govern the earthly triplicity; Cancer, Scorpio, Pisces rule the watery triplicity; and as in the body of Man there are four humors, namely choler, blood, phlegm, and melancholy, so are they represented and governed by the twelve signs according to their several triplicities, for Aries, Leo, Sagittarius are found to be of nature hot and dry, representing choler, Gemini, Libra, Aquarius, hot and moist resembling the blood, Taurus, Virgo, Capricorn cold and dry resembling melancholy, Cancer, Scorpio, Pisces cold and moist representing phlegm. Now, when the principal signs of a disease, or the lord of the sixth house, or the Moon shall be in either of the earthly, airy, fiery or watery signs, judge the quality of the humor offending to be according to their nature, and your judgment will be the more sure, if that the sign of the sixth and lord of the sixth be both of one nature, and posited in a sign of the nature of the sign descending in the sixth house, otherwise we must make an equal commixture, and judge so many humors, offends as are represented by the sign of the sixth house, lord thereof, and sign, wherein the lord of the sixth house, and Moon are posited, as if Aries were in the cusps of the sixth house, and Saturn therein, or the lord of the sixth house, the four elements governed or signified by the twelve signs, and the Moon in Taurus, Virgo, Capricorn especially the lord of the sixth, then we may assuredly resolve, that the disease proceeds from choler and melancholy. Choler, because Aries and Mars lord thereof, are by nature hot and dry representing the choleric humor, melancholy, because Saturn who is by nature cold and dry, representing melancholy is in the sixth house is in a sign representing the same humor, the like may be observed by any other of the signs and Planets, always remembering the former rules, namely, what humor is signified by the sign in the sixth house, and by the lord thereof, and by the planet or Ppanets therein posited, and the sign wherein the lord thereof is placed, and according to their nature judge, making a right commixture as before is shown.

Of the Members in mans body governed by the twelve signs or constellations, and of the diseases signified by them

Aries: The first sign of the Zodiac rules in the body of man, the head, face, eyes, nose, ears, and mouth, and signifies all diseases of a hot and dry nature, incident to those members, as headaches of all sorts, pushes and pimples in the face, all manner of scars in the face.

Taurus: governs the neck, throat and wind-pipe, and has relation unto all diseases of a cold and dry nature, subject unto the throat, the Kings evil, hard kernels or swellings in the neck and throat, congestion, and the like.

Gemini: rules the Arms, hands, shoulders, and all diseases of a hot and moist nature subject to those members are signified by this sign, it hath relation to the blood, and diseases thence arising.

Cancer: Has dominion over the breast, stomach, liver, and lungs, and signifies putrefaction in the stomach, ill digestion, rottenness, and weakness in the stomach, and lungs, all manner of imposthumes, cankers, hurts, or bruises in the breast or stomach.

Leo: Governs the heart, back, ribs and sides, and signifies all hot and dry diseases subject to them, as pleurisy, inflammations, the heart overheated (this is to be understood when Mars is herein) but otherwise it naturally signifies hear problems, fainting, and swooning, and all infirmities incident to the heart.

Virgo: Has the sole power over the bowels, and belly, the small guts and entrails, and has relation unto all diseases coming or arising from wind; it signifies griping in the belly and guts, the colic (but that is when Saturn or Mars shall be author of the disease, and posited in this sign) yet all diseases generally incident to the belly, of a cold and dry nature, as also hardness of dung in the guts, or stopping of the course of the excrement, which we may assuredly judge, if Saturn be author of a disease, and posited in this sign.

Libra: Rules the reins and loins, and has signification of those diseases incident to them, it is of nature hot and moist, representing the blood, and diseases thence arising are attributed to this sign; it also has relation to those diseases subject to the bladder, and naturally signifies all impediments therein, Mars in this sign shows heat of the reins, the stone, rashes and the like infirmities, etc. and sometimes a gonorrhea.

Scorpio: Has signification of diseases in the privy members, in regard they are governed by this sign, naturally it signifies the groin, it also has some relation to the bladder.

Sagittarius: Rules the thighs and hips, and the sciatica, also other infirmities in those parts are signified by this sign, as also the gout, namely the running gout.

Capricorn: Governs the knees, and is of a cold and melancholy nature, all diseases incident to those places, as the leprosy, rashes and scabs in and about the knees, and lower legs, as also all strains or fractures, are attributed to this sign.

Aquarius: Is hot and moist, representing diseases of that nature it resembles the blood, in regard it is an airy sign, it rules in the body of man, the legs and ankles, and signifies all manner of lameness, and bruises in the legs, and all impediments in those members.

Pisces: Is a watery sign, and has dominion over the feet, and the gout and all cold and moist diseases, incident to those members, are signified by this sign, Moon in this sign, and author of the disease, is an assured testimony of the gout in the feet and toes, and swellings in those parts occasioned by cold and moist causes.

THE ASTROLOGICAL PHYSICIAN

What part of the body is afflicted

We must herein consider, first, what sign is in the sixth house, and what member and part of mans body it governs; secondly, in what sign the lord of the sixth is posited, and what part or member that sign represents, in which he is placed: Likewise we must have regard unto the lord of the ascendant, and the Moon, and observe what sign they are in; which being well considered, we shall then find and discover, what part or member of the body is afflicted, but in this we must carefully heed the sign wherein the lord of the sixth is posited, for usually that member governed or signified by that sign, wherein the lord of the sixth is placed, is most afflicted and distempered.

If the Lord of the sixth house be in the ten first degrees of a sign, the upper part of that member, signified by that sign, is most afflicted, if he be in the middle of a sign, the middle of that member signified thereby, is most oppressed, if in the latter part or last degrees of a sign, the lower part of that member represented thereby is most afflicted. As for example, the lord of the sixth house, at the time of the first examination of the sick, or at the time of the propounding of the question in Cancer, in the first part thereof, then we may judge the upper part of the stomach to be afflicted by such diseases as are incident to the upper part thereof, of the nature of the lord of the sixth, the like may be observed by any other sign.

And here we must also observe, that in discovering the nature and quality of any disease, we must not rely only upon the natural signification of the sign, for not the sign only to be considered is enough, but the nature of the planet, who is author of the disease, is principally to be regarded.

THE ASTROLOGICAL PHYSICIAN

Of the Diseases Signified by the Seven Planets, and first of the Diseases signified by the Planet Saturn

Saturn is a planet of nature cold and dry, representing melancholy, all diseases of the like nature are signified by him: all quartian agues, proceeding of cold black jaundices, palsies, consumption, rheumatism, the hand and foot gout, apoplexies, and all infirmities which have their origin from melancholy distempers, are attributed to this planet, he rules in the body of man the spleen.

Now when he shall be author of the disease, or lord of the sixth house, or posited therein, we may judge the sickness to proceed from such causes, as he naturally signifies; but because I would be plain in discussing of the nature of the planets, and of those diseases signified by them, I have thought necessary to insert those infirmities, or diseases, signified by them in any of the twelve signs, therefore observe that which follow:

Saturn in Aries:

When Saturn shall be lord of the sixth house, and posited in Aries, Aries he usually intimates, that the disease arises from melancholy distempers, and that the sick party is much oppressed in the head, and troubled with melancholy vapors there, as also that the sick party is very silent and dull, subject to strange imaginations, fears, and terrible dreams, it has been found by experience, that when Saturn has been author of the disease, and in this sign, that the sick party hath been much afflicted with heaviness in the head, slept very little, but exceedingly troubled with stuffings in the head, sometimes he is oppressed with distillations of rheum from thence, as also with noise and soundings in the head and ears, many times the party is very dull of hearing, and hath great pain in the teeth.

THE ASTROLOGICAL PHYSICIAN

Saturn in Taurus:

When Saturn shall be the sign of the disease, and in Taurus, he creates swellings in the throat, hoarseness, hard kernels there, and many times he gives suspicion of that disease vulgarly called the Kings Evil, he also signifies wens and hard swellings in the neck, and extreme sore throats.

Saturn in Gemini:

Saturn author of the sickness and in Gemini, usually declares all wounds or hurts in the arms or shoulders, but in regard this sign has relation to the blood, therefore we may judge, that when Saturn shall be the sign of a disease, and posited herein, that the blood is too thick, and that the sick party is subject to diseases of a cold, a dry nature, incident to the blood, and sometimes the sick party is inclining to a consumption, or the black jaundices.

Saturn in Cancer:

Saturn principal sign of a disease, and in Cancer, the sick is commonly afflicted with putrefaction in the stomach, the digestive faculty is much weakened, and the sick party is much oppressed with coughs, proceeding from the indisposition of the lungs, commonly it is observed, that the lungs are much decayed for want of moisture; from thence arise many infirmities, sometimes upon this sign the sick party is oppressed with ulceration in the lungs, ptisick, or the like, usually melancholy vapors afflict the stomach and lungs, when Saturn being planet of a disease is posited in this sign, he also signifies cancers, ulcers, and bruises in the breast and stomach, when he shall be found herein.

THE ASTROLOGICAL PHYSICIAN

Saturn in Leo:

Saturn in Leo, and chief author of the disease, declares
the heart to be oppressed with melancholy and stinking vapors,
the sick party is very fretful, and complains usually of great pain
at the heart, many times it has been observed, that when Saturn
has been author of a disease, or principal signification of a
sickness, or infirmity, and posited in this sign, that the sick party
has taken some inward grief, and is much afflicted with
melancholy distempers at the heart, occasioned by too much
sorrow, sometimes poison is to be feared to be the cause of the
sickness, when other testimonies concur.

Saturn in Virgo:

Saturn in Virgo, being lord of the sixth house, and
having most power in a disease, demonstrates that the present
sickness or distemper, proceeds from melancholy obstructions in
the bowels and small guts, commonly and most usually the sick
party is troubled in the belly, the colic is to be feared upon this
position, sometimes I have known when the sick party has been
troubled with illiack passions, and much oppressed with hard
dung in the guts, has gone very seldom to stool: in such a
position as this, let laxative be administered to the sick party.

Saturn in Libra:

Saturn in Libra, and the only signification of a sickness,
or infirmity, commonly intimates great pain in the reins and
bladder: Stoppage of the urine by cold, yet Libra being an airy
sign, the position of Saturn therein may declare some distemper
in the blood, and that the sick parties blood is decaying, and is
thick and windy: moreover when other testimonies agree, the
Strangury is to be feared, as also great pain in the back and
kidneys, whereby the sick party is much oppressed, or some

former bruises.

Saturn in Scorpio:

Saturn in Scorpio, and lord of the sixth house, and author of the disease or infirmity, shows that the sick party is tormented in the privy members, he signifies botches and scabs there, as also bruises, the swellings of those members, and ulcers, in those parts, we may fear upon such a position, that the sick party is troubled with the piles.

Saturn in Sagittarius:

When Saturn shall be signifier as aforesaid, and in the sign of Sagittarius, we have eminent cause to judge, that the sick party is troubled with swellings in the hips, and thighs, pain in those members by cold, old aches, old bruises and the like, and that the infirmity proceeds of some former grief or impediment, however we may mistrust the sciatica in the hips, as also fistulas, and the like soars in those parts.

Saturn in Capricorn, Aquarius, Pisces:

Saturn in Capricorn, and author of the disease, signifies impediment in the knees, lameness and bruises there; yet some do affirm that Saturn, in any of theses signs, which are his houses, namely, Capricorn and Aquarius do represent the head, and so all other planets, when they are in their own houses they do the like, now if Saturn shall be in Aquarius or Pisces, and the signification as aforesaid, then we may judge the sick party to be oppressed with the gout in the feet and toes, and much pain in those members, occasioned through cold distempers in those parts, sometimes the ague, or some other cold disease afflicts the sick party in those members.

THE ASTROLOGICAL PHYSICIAN

We now come to treat of Jupiter, and those diseases signified by him. Jupiter is of nature hot and moist, and represents the blood, and all diseases that have their origin from hot and moist causes, are attributed to this planet, he signifies all diseases, in the liver and lungs, pleurisy, convulsions, inflammations of the liver, apoplexies, windiness in the veins and blood, and all diseases arising from putrefaction there, his signification of diseases in any of the twelve signs is as follows:

Jupiter in Aries:

When Jupiter shall be in Aries, and the principal signification of a disease, he declares that the sickness proceeds of the disaffection of the blood in the head, many times the sick parties face is swelled, and the head much afflicted, usually the temples are red, and the sick party sleeps very poorly, is molested with strange fancies and dreams, usually the cause of the distemper arises from the windiness of the blood, in the veins of the head, sometimes from an inposthume.

Jupiter in Taurus:

Jupiter in Taurus, and signification as aforesaid, gives suspicion of the quinsy, which is a disease usually subject to the throat, however we may judge swellings in that member when we find Jupiter author of the disease, and in this sign, as also that the blood is too thick and dry.

Jupiter in Gemini.:

Jupiter in Gemini, intimates that the disease arises from the overflowing of the blood, and that there is too much, opening of a vein or sweating, is an excellent remedy for such as are afflicted with this infirmity.

THE ASTROLOGICAL PHYSICIAN

Jupiter in Cancer:

Jupiter in Cancer, and principal signification of a disease, shews the blood to be thin and watery, the party inclining to a dropsy, the blood is filled with phlegm, and many times the scurvy and watery humors in the blood, causes the distemper; we may judge also, that the sick party has no great appetite to his victuals, and that his stomach is offended.

Jupiter in Leo:

Jupiter in Leo, intimates, that the disease proceeds of putrefied humors, that the blood is over-heated, the sick party inclining to a fever, which may be confidently affirmed, if other testimonies concur, yet nevertheless the disease has its origin from putrefaction at the heart, bleeding and sweating is much to be commended in this infirmity, for sometimes the disease is pestilential.

Jupiter in Virgo:

Jupiter in Virgo shows the blood to be oppressed, and much infected with melancholy, and that by reason of the coldness and dryness in the liver and lungs, the sick party is much afflicted: many times the flux is to be feared upon this position, however we may judge the blood to be thick, and too gross, and the party inclining to a consumption, in women he signifies fits of the mother.

Jupiter in Libra:

Jupiter in Libra has great signification of the blood, in regard it is an airy sign representing the same, we usually observe upon this position the sick party has great need of bleeding, for the blood abounds exceedingly, from whence sometimes arises corrupt humors, and diseases of putrefaction, many times aduftion of blood, if Venus be with Jupiter in this sign.

Jupiter in Scorpio:

Jupiter in Scorpio has almost the same signification, as in Cancer, only we find that the sick party is more oppressed with salt humors in the blood, we also usually discern some grief in the privy members, in regard this sign hath some relation to them, namely, the Strangury.

Jupiter in Sagittarius, Capricorn, Aquarius, Pisces:

Jupiter in Sagittarius usually denotes choleric humors in the blood, and that it is over-heated by some extravagant exercise, from thence arise fevers proceeding of choler; so likewise, when he is in Capricorn he declares the blood to be afflicted with melancholy, and in Aquarius he intimates that from the abundance of the blood, arises the sickness or infirmity, and also in Pisces he denotes the blood to be watery, and thin, and the dropsy may be feared when Jupiter is in Pisces, and signification of a disease, for the blood is much oppressed with phlegm, and watery humors upon such a posture.

We now in order come to speak of Mars, and the diseases signified by him, but in regard that those diseases attributed to Mars, differ not much from those signified by Sun, in regard they are both of one nature, therefore for brevity's sake, we will handle them both together:

Of the diseases or infirmities signified by Mars and Sun

Mars and Sun: First, Mars is of nature hot and dry, and so likewise Sun, they both represent the choleric humor in man, yet the diseases of Mars, somewhat differ from the diseases signified by Sun: for Mars represents these diseases, and they are wholly attributed to him, because of his violent nature, namely, all imposthumes, burning fevers, the plague, yellow jaundice, all infirmities in the privy members, the bloody flux, all pestilential sores, as fistulas, carbuncles, St. Anthony's fire, calentures, etc. He rules the gall, because it is the receptacle of choler in mans body.

Now the diseases signified by Sun are wounds and heart passions, red choler, cramps, all diseases in general incident to the heart, he signifies the right eye of a man, the left of a woman, the brain is in some part attributed to him, as also the mouth.

The significations of these two planets, and the diseases signified by them, in any of the twelve signs, are as follows: namely:

Mars or Sun in Aries:

When Mars shall be author of a disease, or principal signifier of a sickness, and in Aries, we may judge that the sick party is much tormented in the head, troubled with extreme pain there occasioned, through a hot and dry distemper of the brain, many times the sick party is almost or wholly distracted by reason of choleric humors in the brain, usually the sick party sleeps very little, or not much, in regard of the distemper, sometimes the party is subject to hot rheum in the eyes, and imposthumes in the head, but if Sun be author, as aforesaid, then we may assuredly affirm, that the sick party is perplexed also in the eyes, subject to catarrh, and other infirmities there, however judge the head and brain much distempered, and the sick party almost frantic by reason of the vehemency of the choleric distempers there.

THE ASTROLOGICAL PHYSICIAN

Mars or Sun in Taurus:

Mars Lord of the sixth house, and the only signification of a disease, and posited in Taurus, intimates extreme pain in the neck, pushes or scabs there: also harshness and roughness in the throat and windpipe, and soreness and extreme pain therein, the Kings evil may be mistrusted to be breeding when we find Mars herein. If Sun shall be signification of a disease, and placed in this sign we may judge as aforesaid, and likewise conjecture that the heart is much afflicted with melancholy vapors.

Mars or Sun in Gemini:

Mars in Gemini and signification as I have said before, declares that the sickness or disease comes of heat and dehydration of blood, that the sick party is troubled with the itch or breaking out of humors in the body, bleeding is excellent for the sick, and medicines that cool the blood: For many times the sick party is surfeited by extraordinary heat of the blood, from thence arise pestilential fevers and diseases of putrefaction, by reason of the disaffection of the blood.

Mars and Sun in Cancer:

When Mars shall be principal signification of a disease, and in Cancer, shows that the sick party is very thirsty, and much afflicted by heat in the stomach, and choleric humors there; usually the sick party is much oppressed with pain in the breast and stomach, the lungs are dry and want excrement, namely, phlegm and spittle, the sick party is troubled with a hot and dry cough, many infirmities are in the stomach and lungs, occasioned through choler and phlegm. The like may be judged when the Sun is author of a disease, and posited in this sign; if the question be for a woman, then we may mistrust she has received some hurt in the breast, from thence many times arises cancers, a fistula, or some other rotten putrid sore or imposthume.

Mars and Sun in Leo:

Mars or the Sun in Leo, and either of them author of the disease, or infirmity, intimates that the heart is overheated, and that the sick party is choleric, angry and peevish, occasioned by the vehemency of the hot and dry distemper of the heart; usually upon this position the cause of the sickness proceeds from choler, and that the sick party is much subject to sudden wounds, and heart passions, inclining to a violent fever, or stone in the kidneys.

Mars and Sun in Virgo:

Mars or the Sun, author or chief signification of the sickness, denotes when they shall be posited in Virgo, that the origin of the disease arises of choleric humors in the belly and bowels, most commonly the sick party is oppressed with the colic, which is an infirmity in the gut called colon, the sick party is extraordinarily bound in the body, goes very seldom to stool, much tormented in the bowel by reason of choleric obstructions there, many times bloody flux is to be feared when Mars or the Sun are signs of the disease, and posited in this sign, the worms also in children.

Mars and Sun in Libra:

Mars or the Sun in Libra, either of them being lord of the sixth house, declares that the sick parties blood is much infected with choler, the blood is hot and dry, and much distempered, such things as cool the blood are necessary to be administered to the sick party; however Mars or the Sun, principal signs of a disease, and posited in this sign, shows us, that the sick party is oppressed with a great heat in the reins and kidneys, the stone may be feared upon this position, as also gravel in the urine, the sick party many times has been found to be much tormented in the bladder, the urine very hot, and sometimes the passage thereof stopped, sometimes madness.

Mars and Sun in Scorpio:

Mars of the Sun in Scorpio, and signification as I have said before, intimates great pain in the secret and privy members, extraordinary heat in those parts, this position gives great suspicion of a clap of some unclean woman, and that the disease came that way, if it be a woman that propounds the question, then we may judge that she has used too much the sports of Venus, and she has too great flux of the whites and reds, however we may conjecture of great distempers in those parts which are governed by Scorpio, namely, the secret members, and that the sick party is tormented with some scurvy disease there, perhaps an ulcer.

Mars and Sun in Sagittarius:

When the Sun or Mars shall be either of them in Sagittarius and Lord of the sixth house, or significations of a disease, judge the sick to be afflicted in the hips and thighs, through pestilent and choleric humors in those parts, fistula's or terrible sores there, or a sciatica.

Mars and Sun in Capricorn, Aquarius, Pisces:

Now Mars or the Sun in Capricorn, Aquarius and Pisces, and author of the infirmity as aforesaid, declares the distemper to arise from choleric humors, descending into the knees, legs, and feet, many times they signify scabs and sores in those members, when there are other testimonies of the same, they signify also lameness in those parts, many times the joint gout.

Of the Diseases signified by Venus and the Moon

Venus and Moon:

Venus and Luna are both of one nature, namely, cold and moist, and so are the diseases attributed to them, the diseases and infirmities signified by Venus are these, namely suffocation, all defections in the matrix, weakness in the act of generation, debility and weakness in the stomach, gonorrhea, the French Pox, she rules the sperm or seed in man or woman.

Luna signifies the falling sickness, palsies, menses in Women, aposthumes, looseness in the belly, cold and raw humors in any part of the body, dropsy, gout, surfeit, rotten coughs, apoplexies, rheums in the eyes, she rules the left eye of men, and the right eye of women. Now in regard Venus and Moon are both of one nature, we will therefore treat of them both together, as we did of Sun and Mars the diseases signified by Venus or the Moon in any of the twelve signs, are as follows:

Venus and Moon in Aries:

Venus or the Moon in Aries, and signs of the disease or infirmity, declare that the sick party is molested with cold humors in the head, troubled with too much rheum there, the brain is too cold and moist, the sick parties' senses are very dull, abundance of excrement flows from the brain, usually the sickness proceeds of cold, and the sick is very desirous of sleep, his head is stuffed with rheum, and the sick party very heavy, lethargy, coma carus, and other diseases of the head that proceed of cold and moisture, may be feared by the physician.

Venus and Moon in Taurus:

Venus or the Moon in Taurus, and signifier, either of them as aforesaid, intimate raw humors in the neck, swellings there, by reason of abundance of moisture flowing from the head; there usually upon this position, some cold rheum in the neck, or cold swellings there, whereby the sick party is distempered.

Venus and Moon in Gemini:

Venus or Luna author of the disease, and in Gemini, denotes that the blood is oppressed with watery humors, the dropsy may be feared upon this position, and other diseases of that nature, the veins are full of watery blood, and it is very necessary to correct the cold and moist distemper of the blood, for from thence doth the sickness arise: the sick party is very faint and weak usually, and subject to swellings in the arms, and divers other places in the body.

Venus and Moon in Cancer:

Venus or Luna in Cancer, and principal signifier of the disease, declare that the sickness proceeds of cold and raw matter in the stomach, the sick party has little appetite to victuals, but is molested with rheum, and cold and watery humors in the stomach, phlegm abounds much there, and the sick is much perplexed with straining to vomit, and all the distemper in the stomach, arises from too much moisture there.

Venus and Moon in Leo:

Venus and Luna signifier, either of them as aforesaid, and in Leo, acquaints us that the origin of the disease proceeds of cold and moist vapors at the heart, but seldom any great distemper happens upon this position, in regard the heart is more afflicted by the position of Saturn or Mars in this sign, then by any other planet.

Venus and Moon in Virgo:

When Venus or Luna is in Virgo, and either of them signifier of a disease, we may judge that the sick party is much troubled with raw humors in the bowels and guts, from whence comes a looseness or flux of the belly, many times it has been found that the sick party has been oppressed, and tormented with worms, and much afflicted by often going to stool, occasioned by cold and slimy humors in the belly and guts.

Venus and Moon in Libra:

Venus or Luna in Libra, and either of them author of the disease or sickness, tells us that the sick party is surfeited by over much drinking and eating, it sometimes happens, that the sick party is much troubled with the gonorrhea, or running of the urine, the diabetes or pissing disease, any disease arising by inordinate lust, is signified by this position, for Venus naturally governs and signifies such diseases, and being sign of a disease, and in this sign, imports weakness in the urine, yet we may judge the blood also to be too thin, and filled with phlegm and water, in regard it is an airy sign.

Venus and Moon in Scorpio:

Venus or the Moon in Scorpio, and either of them signification of a sickness or disease, intimates that the origin of the distemper or infirmity, comes of too much use of lustful actions, usually the sick party is troubled much in the privy members, for the which he may thank his own folly, if a woman demands the question for herself, or if it be propounded for a female party, then judge that she has been too familiar with men: however we may conjecture upon this position, that the sickness is occasioned by too much lust, and by the common and too frequent use of those members represented by this sign, many times the stones are swelled.

Venus and Moon in Sagittarius:

Moon or Venus signification of a disease in Sagittarius, declares the gout or swellings in the thighs, the hips, gout, or sciatica may be feared, botches and sores in the hips and thighs, cold and moist humors being the cause thereof.

Venus and Moon in Capricorn, Aquarius, Pisces:

Venus or the Moon signification as aforesaid, and in either of these signs, namely, Capricorn, Aquarius, or Pisces, shows and signifies the gout in the knees and feet: swellings in the legs through cold anguished humors, there the gout or dropsical humors may be feared to be the cause of the sickness of infirmity, when Venus or Moon are significations, and in either of these signs.

Of the Diseases signified by the Planet Mercury

Although in order Mercury ought to have been treated of before the Moon, yet in regard Venus and Moon were both of one nature, we held it convenient to treat of both their significations together, in any of the twelve signs, therefore we now come to speak of Mercury, and of the diseases signified by him. Mercury is a Planet of nature cold and dry, representing melancholy; yet he is of a variable nature, for his influence is usually according to the nature of the planet, with the which he is conjoined; the diseases signified by him are these, namely, all such as proceed of cold and wind, vertigo, lethargy, giddiness in the head, madness or lightness, or any other disease adherent to the brain, all stammering or imperfection in the tongue, defects in the memory, hoarseness or dry coughs, ptisick, all evils in the intellectual parts, etc. He has principal relation to the brain, tongue, lungs and memory. The diseases or infirmities signified by Mercury, in any of the twelve signs are as follows:

Mercury in Aries:

When Mercury shall be the principal author of a disease or sickness, and in Aries, he shows that the sick party is much troubled with wind in the head, and brain, yet the memory is pretty good, the sick party is almost giddy, and complains of lightness in the head, talks sometimes idly, and if Mercury be with Mars in this sign the party is almost distracted, if with Saturn, he stammers much in speaking, such things as dispel wind and comfort the animal spirits, and open obstructions, are necessary to be administered in this infirmity.

Mercury in Taurus:

Mercury in Taurus, and signification as aforesaid, acquaints us with hard kernels in the neck, stiffness there, as also hoarseness in the Throat, and roughness in the windpipe, strangulation and wheezing there.

Mercury in Gemini:

Mercury in Gemini, and signification of the disease, shows windiness in the veins and blood.

Mercury in Cancer:

Mercury in Cancer, and principal signification as aforesaid, intimates the stomach to be oppressed with cold and wind, the sick party troubled with sour belching, and griping there, continual pain by wind.

Mercury in Leo:

Mercury in Leo, and author of the disease, declares the heart to be oppressed with melancholy, as also the sick party to be tormented with pain and shootings in the back, and at the heart.

Mercury in Virgo.:

Mercury in Virgo, and signification as aforesaid, expresses the bowels to be tormented with wind, the sick party much oppressed in the belly, great pain therein, the wind colic usually afflicts the sick party upon this position.

Mercury in Libra:

Mercury in Libra, and author of the disease, tells us that the blood is windy, great pain in the reins by cold, the urine stopped by reason of the pain in the reins and bladder, the urine usually is very windy and frothy.

Mercury in Scorpio:

Mercury in Scorpio, hath no great signification, only declares pain in the privy members by cold, as also windiness in those parts.

Mercury in Sagittarius, Capricorn, Aquarius, Pisces:

Mercury in Sagittarius, Capricorn, Aquarius, or Pisces denote windy and cold swellings in those members signified by those signs.

THE ASTROLOGICAL PHYSICIAN

Thus have I as plainly as possible may be, given you the seven planets, in any of the twelve signs, being lord or ruler of the sixth house, or principal signification of the disease or sickness; I might now proceed to speak of the signification of the aspects of the planets one with another, especially of the Moon, for we must diligently observe what planet she is in configuration with, and what planet the lord of the ascendant, and Lord of the sixth house are in configuration with, in what sign, the nature and quality of the sign, and nature of the Aspect, and accordingly we are to judge; but in regard I have been so plain in my former rules, I think it not expedient to treat of the aspects, by reason we may easily judge of the signification of the configurations of the planets, one with the other, in any of the twelve signs, by the foregoing rules, ever remembering the nature of the planet, in configuration with the lord of the ascendant, lord of the sixth house, or the Moon, and according to his nature judge, making a right commixture as I have formerly said. I will now speak somewhat concerning the ascendant and lord thereof.

First therefore, we must observe what sign ascends, and the nature of the lord of the ascendant, and sign wherein he is, are to be considered, for it signifies much in this manner of judgment, the ascendant represents the head and face, it declares the sick parties complexion, it further intimates whether the brain is disturbed or not, or whether the disease lies more in the mind then in the body,, that is, it shows whether the parties senses be troubled or oppressed more then any part of the body, the signification of any of the seven planets in the ascendant, is as follows:

When Saturn shall be in the ascendant afflicted, and chief signification of the disease, and he is not lord of the ascendant, then we may judge that the sick party is much afflicted in the head with melancholy vapors, is silent, speaks very little, complains of great noise and stuffings in the head, and ears, usually if Saturn be in the ascendant, the sick parties head and brain is much distempered.

Jupiter as lord of the sixth house, or principal signification of the disease, and in the ascendant or first house, declares that the head and face is much oppressed by hot and moist humors flowing thither, occasioned by too much blood, the sick party has a very high color, and many times the veins in the temples are swelled, and likewise in the face also, this distemper afflicts the sick party most, when the wind is South.

Mars the signification as aforesaid, and he not lord of the ascendant, and posited accidentally therein, shows that the sick party is perplexed in the head by choleric humors, is also much troubled in the brain, almost frenetic, and molested with extreme pain in the head, sleeps very poorly nor is the sick much subject to sleep, when Mars is in the ascendant, by reason of the hot and dry distemper of the brain.

Sun signification or author of the disease, and in the ascendant, usually signifies the same that Mars does, only sometimes the sick party is troubled with terrible sore eyes, and inflammations therein, or cataracts, a disease which usually takes away the sight.

Venus and the Moon in the ascendant, and either of them signification as aforesaid, tells us that the sick party is stuffed in the head by cold, troubled with rheum in the head and eyes, occasioned by the cold and moistness of the brain, from thence arises apoplexies, the falling sickness, palsies, lethargy, coma Carus, and other diseases incident to the head and brain, proceeding of cold and moist humors.

Mercury in the first house, and author of sickness, as I

have said before, intimates that the sick parties head is much distempered by wind and cold, and the brain is also much afflicted by the same, the sick party is also very giddy and light headed subject to vertigo and the like diseases; also Cauda draconis in the ascendant signifies much distemper in the head.

By what has been delivered, the physician may now suddenly and most easily find the nature and quality of a disease or sickness by the heavens, which is the only way, and most assured for discovering of the quality of the humor offending in any disease, as Galen, Hippocrates, and the first founders of the art of medicine affirm.

Now what has been said concerning the position of the signification of the disease in the ascendant, the like may also be observed by the position of the lord of the sixth house, or author of the disease, in any of the other houses; for as the first house or ascendant signifies the head and face, so do the other houses signify these several parts or members in mans body:

> The second house signifies Neck and Throat.
> The third, Arms, Hands, and Shoulders.
> The fourth, Breast, Stomach and Lungs.
> The fifth, Liver, heart, Sides and Back.
> The sixth, the Belly and Bowels.
> The seventh, the Haunches, and Navel to the Buttocks.
> The eight, the Bladder and privy parts.
> The ninth, the Hips and Thighs.
> The tenth, the Knees and Hams.
> The eleventh, the Legs and Ankles.
> The twelfth, the Feet.

Having now plainly shown how to discover the nature of any disease, and judge upon any distemper, the quality and cause thereof in a natural way, we hold it in the next place convenient to declare how to find out the short and long continuance of any sickness or disease, for the which observe the succeeding method.

Whether the sickness will be short or of long continuance

If we desire to know how long the sickness will continue, we must consider and carefully observe what sign is in the sixth house, and what planet is author of the disease, or principal signification, for those diseases or infirmities signified by Saturn, are long and permanent by reason of his slowness; diseases signified by Mars or Sun, are very short, although terrible, Jupiter also signifies short diseases, and Venus a mean betwixt both, Mercury, such as are inconstant, and Moon signifies sudden change, and alteration of the disease, either for better or worse; moreover the sign, as I have said before, which is in the sixth house, and in which the signification is posited, are also to be regarded, for some signs are movable, some fixed, and some are common, the movable are, Aries, Cancer, Libra, Capricorn, fixed signs are these; Taurus, Scorpio, Leo, Aquarius. Common signs are, Gemini, Virgo, Sagittarius, Pisces. Now if we find a movable sign in the sixth house, and the lord thereof, and the Moon or principal signification of the disease in a movable sign, then we may judge the sickness to be short, if they shall be in fixed signs, judge long and tedious sickness, but if they be in common signs, judge a mediocrity, and that the disease will neither be too short or long, but that you may be better instructed in this, observe these Aphorisms.

First: Lord of the sixth, in the sixth, signifies a durable and tedious sickness.

Second: Lord of the sixth house in square or opposition to the ascendant, or applying to the lord thereof, argues the same, and that the disease is not in its full force and power.

THE ASTROLOGICAL PHYSICIAN

Third: The lord of the sixth retrograde signifies a relapse.

Fourth: The lord of the sixth house removing out of one sign into another, and also the latter degrees of any sign, upon the cusps of the sixth house, denotes sudden change, and alteration of the disease.

Fifth: The Lord of the ascendant in the sixth house, or the Lord of the sixth in the ascendant, intimates a great sickness, and of long continuance, if they be in fixed signs.

Sixth: And lastly, if the principal signification of the disease, be in movable signs, judge a sudden change of the disease, if they be in fixed signs or common, judge as aforesaid.

If the sick party shall recover from his sickness or not

In resolving this question, we are to consider the strength of the Lord of the ascendant, and what favorable aspect is cast unto him, and we are to see if there be any benevolent planet in the ascendant, for if Jupiter or Venus who are naturally Fortunes, shall be in the ascendant, or with the lord thereof in a good house of Heaven, and they not lords of the sixth, eighth, or twelfth houses, then we may judge nature is strong, so likewise if the lord of the ascendant be free from misfortune, essentially strong and more powerful, then the Lord of the sixth house, it is a good sign, for nature seems then to be more strong, and better fortified then the disease, and also able to work out the offending humor.

Moreover if the lord of the ascendant be free from any aspect of the Lord of the eight house, or planet posited in the eight, and also free from combustion, and not under the sun beams, it is a strong argument of recovery, likewise if there be no translation of light between the lord of the eighth, and lord of the ascendant, and if the Moon be free from any aspect of the lord of the eighth house, or planet posited therein, then it signifies good to the sick party, and gives hopes of recovery.

The lord of the tenth house being in a friendly aspect with the lord of the ascendant, argues that the sick party shall be cured by medicine, the like signification has Jupiter or Venus, being in the ascendant, or with the lord thereof. Now it is to be noted, that the seventh house represents the physician, the tenth house his medicine, if therefore the seventh house be afflicted, the physician shall not cure the sick party, if the tenth house be also afflicted, the physic which has been, or is administered to the sick, is not proper for the disease, and works no good effect.

Testimonies of Death

The most assured argument of the death of the sick party, is when the lord of the eighth house is in the ascendant, or with the lord thereof, for if the lord of the eighth house shall be in the ascendant, we may justly fear the death of the sick, so likewise if any planet in the eighth house afflict the ascendant, or lord thereof, death may be feared; also if any planet translate the light or influence of the lord of the eighth, or planet in the eighth, to the lord of the ascendant, then it is an ill omen, and of dangerous consequence to the sick party.

The lord of the sixth house in the eighth, and afflicting the lord of the ascendant, or translating the virtue and influence of the lord of the eighth, or principal signification of death, to the lord of the ascendant, then we may mistrust and fear that the disease will kill the sick party, and that death is at hand; likewise if the Moon shall be afflicted by the lord of the eighth house, or signification of death, or translate the virtue of the lord of the eighth, to the lord of the ascendant, then the disease is mortal.

When the Lord of the ascendant is in conjunction with

the lord of the eighth, or in square or opposition of him or any planet posited in that house, without the benevolent trine or sextile of Jupiter or Venus intervening declares death.

The lord of the ascendant combust in the eighth, imports the death of the sick, and if also the lord of the ascendant, shall be in the fourth house, in conjunction with the lord of the eighth, we may confidently affirm, that the sick party will die, in regard the signification of life is then afflicted by the lord of the eighth Subterranean.

When the lord of the ascendant also shall be Cadent, and the lord of the sixth angular, then we may judge a terrible strong sickness.

The most assured rules to be observed in pronouncing death of the sick, are these: Lord of the ascendant in the eighth, afflicted, or lord of the eighth in the ascendant, or the Moon in the eighth, applying to the lord of the ascendant by square or opposition, or any other planet in the eighth, in the like configuration with the Lord of the ascendant, the ascendant also afflicted by the presence of any fixed star, of a violent influence of the nature of the lord of the eighth house.

These positions and configurations, or any of them, are I say assured testimonies of the death of the sick party, for whom the question is demanded.

Now if we desire to be resolved, how long it will be before the death of the sick party, if we find testimony of death, as aforesaid, then we must observe how many degrees are between the lord of the eighth, and lord of the ascendant, or between the planet posited in the eighth, applying to the lord of the ascendant, or what number of degrees are before the lord of the ascendant, or the Moon, are in perfect conjunction, square, or many months from the time of the question, but if the aspect be in movable signs, judge so many days as they are distant in degrees from their true aspects, in common signs so many weeks, making a right observation from every signification, for not upon one bare testimony doe we pronounce death, but when we find those assured rules previously delivered, do manifest the same opposition of the principal signification of death, or Lord of the eighth house; if the planet who is signification of death as aforesaid, be in the ascendant, observe then how many degrees he wants of the cusps of the house, and likewise further have regard to the Lord of the ascendant, if he be going to combustion, or under the Sun beams, and note how many degrees are between the Sun and him, before they come to their perfect conjunction, for if they be in movable signs, then so many degrees, as they are distant one from the other, denotes so many days, it will be before the sick party dies.

If the signification of death shall be in a common sign, and the lord of the ascendant also in a common sign, afflicted by the lord of the eighth by any aspect, then it denotes so many weeks as are degrees between their conjunction or aspect; so likewise in fixed signs they denote months, as for example, admit the lord of the eighth house to be hastening to conjunction of the lord of the ascendant, or the lord of the ascendant applying to him by any aspect, and they in fixed signs, and at the time of the propounding of the question for the sick party, distant from each other, 1, 2, 3, or 4 degrees or more, then we may judge the death of the sick, after such a time.

Having now plainly shown how to judge upon any disease happening according to natural causes, we hold not amiss to discover the right way in finding out, whether the disease be natural or not, namely, if the sick party be sick or distempered by such diseases as are incident to mankind, or is bewitched. When the question shall be so demanded for the sick, observe that which follows:

If the sick party be bewitched or not

When it shall be demanded whether one be bewitched or not, then have regard to the lord of the twelfth house, and observe whether he be in any malevolent aspect of the lord of the ascendant, or posited in the ascendant, for if the lord of the twelfth afflicts the ascendant or lord thereof, either by his corporal presence, or by square or opposition aspects, or if they be afflicted or oppressed by any malevolent planet in the twelfth, then the sickness or disease is more then natural: likewise the lord of the ascendant in the twelfth, argues the same; but in delivering judgment upon this query, observe these aphorisms.

First: If the ascendant shall be oppressed by the lord of the twelfth, or the lord thereof, afflicted in the twelfth, then it is to be feared, the sick party is bewitched.

Second: The Moon in the twelfth, or any other planet therein in opposition to the lord of the ascendant, argues that an evil spirit has power over the sick party.

Third: Lord of the ascendant combust in the twelfth, intimates the same.

Fourth: Lord of the ascendant in the sixth, in opposition, to the Lord of the twelfth house, gives suspicion of witchcraft.

Fifth: Lord of the ascendant also, lord of the twelfth, and unfortunate, declares that the sick party is under an ill tongue, so likewise the sign of the ascendant, and sign of the twelfth both one, intimate the same.

Sixth: The lord of the eighth in the twelfth, or applying

to the lord thereof, and then immediately joining to the lord of the ascendant, translating thereby the influence of the twelfth house, and lord thereof, to the ascendant, signifies the death of the sick party by witchcraft.

Seventh: The lord of the sixth house, in the eighth, twelfth, or sixth, signifies a secret and occult disease, more then natural.

These aphorisms, they signify and declare the most approved and assured way in judging of witchcraft.

Now in judging or discovering what party it is that bewitches the sick, or has enchanted him, then describe the planet that is lord of the twelfth house, and you shall have the complexion, stature, and condition of the witch, ever considering in what house of heaven he is posited, and out of what house he afflicts the ascendant, or lord thereof, and what house he is lord of besides the twelfth, so shall you have with due consideration, the cause of the Witches enchanting the sick party.

Lord of the third, lord also of the twelfth , or posited therein, or afflicting the ascendant, or lord thereof, or lord of the twelfth in the third house, afflicting the ascendant, or lord thereof, shows the witch to be a near neighbor to the sick party, etc. and so if we consider in what house the lord of the twelfth is in, and out of what house he afflicts the lord of the ascendant, we shall have also the cause of enchantment.

Of the true crisis or Critical and Judicial days

The true crisis is found out by the motion of the Moon, namely, by her square and opposite place to the sign, degree and minute in which she was placed at the parties first falling sick, therefore for finding the exact crisis, or critical days, observe these ensuing rules.

First: At the time of the parties first falling sick, let the place of the Moon be exactly rectified: note in what sign, degree, and minute of the zodiac she is then placed.

Second: Observe when she comes to the square thereof, for that is the first crisis.

Third: When the Moon comes to her true opposition, that is, to the opposite place in the which she was at the parties first falling sick, then is the second crisis.

Fourth: When she comes to the next square, it is the third crisis.

Fifth: When the Moon hath run round the Heavens, and comes to the very same sign, degree and minute, in the which she was placed at the time of the parties first falling sick, it is the fourth crisis.

Now the judicial days are the middle between the two crisis, there may be discerned also an alteration of the disease, of sudden change thereof, when the Moon comes to be distant from her true place, at the time of the parties first falling sick forty five degrees, so likewise when she is distant ninety degrees, and also when she is distant one hundred thirty five degrees: And as the crisis is the sudden change of the disease, or alteration for better or worse, in other words, trending either to health, or a further sickness, so the days critical, and decretory, show a more certain and sure judgment, whereby the physician may fully discern which way the disease will tend, or whereby the crisis may be exactly judged, for the decretory or critical days, declares a more sure judgment of the infirmity afflicting, namely, whether it will be more powerful, or in a smaller measure at those times,

THE ASTROLOGICAL PHYSICIAN

when the exact crisis is, for when the crisis is, there is a sharp contention betwixt nature and the disease, and if at the time of this crisis, nature is more prevalent then the disease, it is then a good sign; but on the contrary, if the sickness prevails, then the crisis is dangerous, but I shall leave the prosecution of these things until some other opportunity be offered- only by the way, observe these Aphorisms.

First: Then seeing that it is most certain that the Moon by her motion shows the true crisis, and that also the judicial or critical days are found out by her motion in the zodiac, then we must be sure to have regard how she is disposed, whether fortunate or unfortunate, and how she is aspected by the benevolent planets, or the malevolent or malignant planets. And further observe, at the time of the true crisis, whether she be in configuration with the lord of the sixth house, or Lord of the eighth, for if she shall be at the time of the crisis in any malevolent aspect of the lord of the sixth, it is an ill sign, so likewise if she shall be afflicted by the lord of the eighth, it gives great cause to judge the death of the sick party upon that crisis.

Second: If she be then going to the square or opposition of the lord of the sixth, the disease and sickness increases, if she be fortunately aspected at the time of the crisis, by Jupiter or Venus, and they not lords of the sixth, eighth, or twelfth houses, it is a good crisis.

Third: The Moon transiting the cusps of the sixth, eighth, or twelfth, at the time of the crisis, death or prolongation of the disease is to be feared.

Fourth: In Judicial days, the Moon fortunate and well aspected, declares a good crisis to be expected, but if she be unfortunate, she declares the contrary.

THE ASTROLOGICAL PHYSICIAN

Some think that the seventh and fourteenth days are critical, and that these days after the first falling sick of the party, are the first and second crisis, which is a very absurd opinion, in regard that the critical and decretory days proceed not from inferior causes, as some men think, for the learned will observe, that the Moon has great influence and dominion upon our inferior bodies; whereby the humors are stirred up by her motion, so that thereby the true crisis of the disease is declared, and in regard the Moon sometimes moves very swiftly, and again at other times very slowly, being many times inconstant in her motion, therefore she makes the true crisis, not every seventh day, as many conceive: but of these matters I shall have occasion in another treatise hereafter to speak more copiously thereof, therefore at present let the former rules suffice.

THE END

www.ingramcontent.com/pod-product-compliance
Lightning Source LLC
Chambersburg PA
CBHW072033230526
45468CB00021B/1683